Dr. Jim's Guide to Avoiding a Prostate Nightmare

James Occhiogrosso

Published by James Occhiogrosso, 2021.

While every precaution has been taken in the preparation of this book, the publisher assumes no responsibility for errors or omissions, or for damages resulting from the use of the information contained herein.

DR. JIM'S GUIDE TO AVOIDING A PROSTATE NIGHTMARE

First edition. July 31, 2021.

Copyright © 2021 James Occhiogrosso.

ISBN: 979-8201481117

Written by James Occhiogrosso.

Also by James Occhiogrosso

Solutions for Erectile Dysfunction
Your Prostate, Your Libido, Your Life
Dr. Jim's Guide to the Aging Male Body
Dr. Jim's Guide to Avoiding a Prostate Nightmare

Table of Contents

Dr. Jim's Guide To Avoiding a Prostate Nightmare

James Occhiogrosso, N.D.

A Guide to Understanding How Urologists Have Misled Men into Losing Their Prostates and their Sexuality For the Past Thirty Years!

Copyright© 2021 by James Occhiogrosso, N.D.

Written and Published by James Occhiogrosso.

This is copyrighted material. All rights reserved worldwide. This book is free of any copy protection or encryption and is licensed to the original purchaser for his/her personal enjoyment only. If you are reading this book and did not buy it, please respect the Author's rights by buying your own copy and not copying any part of this book for someone else. Thank you for respecting the hard work and rights of this Author.

This book is not meant to substitute for qualified medical advice from a professional. While many of the recommendations are based on common sense, serious concerns are best addressed by a competent medical practitioner.

While every precaution has been taken to assure accuracy in the preparation of this book, the author assumes no responsibility for errors or omissions, or for damages resulting from the use of the information contained herein.

Cover photo by: JC Gellidon

Prolog

One of the quotes medical students hear about on their way to becoming doctors is attributed to the ancient Greek physician Hippocrates. It is typically known as the Hippocratic oath. Quoted from his writings is the term "*primum non nocere.*" Its translation from Latin to English is "First, do no harm." Some medical schools ask their graduates to abide by this oath and others do not.

Unfortunately, many medical doctors tend to minimize the side effects of the procedures they perform or the medications they prescribe. When a man encounters typical symptoms of aging and reports them to his doctor, he is often subject to investigative procedures that can have significant deleterious effects on his life.

While a man may not specifically mention sexuality subjects to his doctor, he can easily be devastated if a procedure for his prostate results in complete sexual inadequacy for life. This is often the case with men treated for prostate cancer and other prostate problems. Unfortunately, in many cases, the damage done by a procedure and sometimes medications cannot be overcome.

While prostate cancer can indeed be a serious medical issue, it is a well-known fact, documented in peer-to-peer medical journals, that prostate cancer and other prostate conditions are highly subject to overdiagnosis and overtreatment. And, in many cases the overtreated patient is left with little recourse for recovering his devastated sexual ability.

As a natural health practitioner for many years, I have been witness to this devastation multiple times. I am hopeful this book will save a few men from "A Prostate Nightmare."

Introduction

As an older guy that has dealt with prostate issues for the past 25 or so years; As a young man who lost his 52 YO father to a botched prostate surgery; As a natural health practitioner for the past twenty or so years that has helped hundreds of men with prostate problems; And, as a doctor of Naturopathy – whose main practice consists of men over 60. I guess I am uniquely qualified to write a book like this one.

For many years, I have been privileged to advise men about their various prostate issues. I worked with some of them to resolve their issues and sent others off to the urological community when their problems were of a nature that I was not competent to deal with.

When I started as a natural health practitioner, I billed myself as a prostate specialist, with both a book and a website devoted to prostate problems. Almost all of my initial clients were men with various prostate or sexual problems. The clients that I helped often tried to get their friends with similar problems in to see me. Regretfully, I rarely saw a friend of one of my clients as a client.

Men are strange animals. While they can easily accept advice from another guy at the gym, it is difficult for them to accept a recommendation to see a specific doctor. Perhaps it is because men are – as I said above – strange animals. I guess too, that taking advice from a practitioner that works out of a home office, is not a medical doctor, and does not wear a white coat or a stethoscope around his neck is taboo.

Anyway, it saddens me in a way, especially when a client that I have specifically helped recommends someone, and he never calls me. One guy that I helped considerably had been going to a local urologist that diagnosed him with all kinds of problems, including bladder and prostate cancer. After several visits with him and getting an extensive history, I told him he was unlikely to have the problems his urologist said he did, (bladder and prostate cancer) and I sent him to visit a very thorough urologist I knew.

It was determined his urinary issues were not due to cancer, but rather, due to s serious case of Benign Prostate Hyperplasia or BPH, a very common malady of older men. He did not need surgery or radiation, he needed some herbal supplements – the kind they have been using in Europe and the rest of the world for treating BPH for many years.

Within a few months he was waking once per night to urinate instead of the 3 to 4 times he was used to. His sexual activity has improved considerably and his overall health is much better.

He told numerous friends about how I have helped him, but he summed up the reaction of his friends when he told me that one of the guys at his golf club said to him, "I've been seeing the same urologist for 20 years, why should I change now?"

Well, several years later, his friend, well into his 80's succumbed to a problem as he submitted to surgery to remove his so-called cancerous prostate. The problem resulted in his subsequent death. This brings to light two facts that should have been take into account pror to recommending surgery. His friend was nearly 90 years old and in poor health. In my opinion, the only reason he was having surgery was that his doctor insisted on it. At his age and considering his co-morbidities, it seems very unlikely that the surgery was justified. But then, this is my not-so-humble opinion.

The book, "Invasion of the Prostate Snatchers" by Mark Scholz, M.D. and Ralph Blum should be required reading for any man with prostate issues. Dr. Scholz is a board-certified medical oncologist, and Mr. Blum a long-time prostate cancer survivor that lived with his prostate cancer for more that 20 years. Mr. Blum passed in 2016 at the age of 84.

As of this writing, Dr. Scholz continues to serve as medical director of Prostate Oncology Specialists Inc. in Marina del Rey, CA. He is also the Executive Director of the Prostate Cancer Research Institute.

I WROTE THIS BOOK IN the hope that I can save a few guys from having surgery, radiation or other treatment that they do not really need. Many doctors that treat prostate issues are in denial of the side effects of either the procedures they perform or the medications they prescribe. Some of them are also more swayed by profit motivations more than their concern for their patients.

Since the PSA test was introduced about three decades ago, the number of men receiving a prostate cancer diagnosis has skyrocketed. However, the methods used to diagnose this potentially serious condition have evolved very little. This is a real problem! It should have been be addressed by the medical/urological community years ago but it continues to linger today.

> Typical of much of the medical community, once a procedure has become ingrained it often takes decades to phase it out, even when it is of dubious value. As an outrageous example of this, the procedure of "bloodletting" – the withdrawal of blood from a patient to cure illness, – is said to have originated in ancient Egypt more than 2000 years ago. While the practice is no longer widespread today, bloodletting persisted into the 20th century and according to Wikipedia, was recommended in the 1923 edition of the textbook "*The Principles and Practice of Medicine.*"[1]

Prostate surgery leaves behind some devastating side effects. Other treatments for prostate cancer can have similar devastating side effects. With the exception of "Watchful Waiting" or "Active Surveillance" All treatments for prostate cancer have serious and devastating side effects, regardless of what your doctor tells you.

A word here on "Watchful Waiting" or "Active Surveillance". In my opinion, they are the same. Both refer to a process whereby a diagnosed case of prostate cancer is periodically evaluated for progression with various tests but without aggressive treatment. However, depending on the specific doctor's approach, this can vary from a regular PSA test, to a full-blown periodic analysis and prostate biopsy.

Almost universally, the men that come to me after medical treatment are hoping I can do the impossible, i.e. recover the function they lost due to aggressive treatment. Unfortunately, my magic wand is not that good! I cannot undo permanent side effects of various medications, nor can I restore function that has been destroyed by the surgical knife.

Many of the men I consulted with came to me because their doctor had tested their PSA and the result was higher than the published norm. In most cases, my advice was to wait a couple weeks and retest. Those that followed this advice often found that the retest measured their PSA in the normal range with no further action needed. Others went on for a biopsy and were diagnosed with prostate cancer. Most of them subsequently had their prostates surgically removed.

Some men were told they had prostate cancer and would die without treatment. Many agreed to surgery simply because of fear. Deep down they knew that overdiagnosis and overtreatment were potentially possible, but their ingrained fear of cancer often led them to an emotional point where they could no longer function effectively.

It is nearly impossible to diagnose a man with prostate cancer and then direct him to an approach like watchful waiting or active surveillance. Many in our society look at anything other then an aggressive treatment plan as "taking no action". It is easier to tell a man he has cancer and it will be treated shortly with surgery, even though his doctor knows the surgery may not really be needed.

Also, in our current environment, treatment is often a more acceptable option. Men who were well-informed better understood what they were facing and were more amicable to researching their options rather than succumbing to immediate surgery.

About The Prostate

The prostate is a walnut-sized gland positioned in the lower abdomen just below the urinary bladder. The gland surrounds the main tube that passes through the penis called the urethra that carries urine out of the body. The prostate's primary purpose is to provide seminal fluid for the male ejaculate during sexual intercourse. It is also the seat of a man's sexual pleasure and ability and provides the pleasurable contractions during intercourse and orgasm.

A properly functioning prostate gland and its associated nerve bundles are essential for sexual function. When the prostate malfunctions, all sorts of symptoms arise, including erectile dysfunction, inability to reach an orgasm, pain on arousal or orgasm, and various urinary problems.

Most men do not know much about the prostate and pay little attention to it as long as it is working fine. However, they suddenly focus their attention on it when it starts to cause problems. The problems it causes are typically age related, and many men tend to view them as inevitable. But, when a doctor starts talking about the possibility of cancer, they usually are "all ears!"

The prostate is the only organ in the body that tends to grow with aging. This growth results in a condition that is common among older men called Benign Prostate Hypertrophy or BPH. The critical word here is *benign.* It is defined by the American Cancer Society (ACS) as: "A growth that is not cancer. It does not invade nearby tissue or spread to other parts of the body."

Benign can also refer to a tumor that is not cancerous. A benign tumor can grow quite large and be found near blood vessels, around the brain, nerves, or organs, but it does not exhibit the uncontrolled cell division that is characteristic of cancer.

Several prominent medical researchers have labeled some prostate tumors as indolent prostate cancer. The term indolent is defined by the National Institute of Health (NIH) as a "potentially inconsequential malignancy inherent to cancer screening. It can often be a cancer that would not become symptomatic in a patient's lifetime and would not contribute to death."

A recent study (see next section) of men that died from causes other than prostate cancer (stroke, heart attack, accident) concluded that prostate anomalies were found at a rate that was nearly equivalent to the man's age in percent. Or, in other words a 70 YO man had about a 70 percent chance of having undiagnosed or indolent prostate cancer.

Thus, while few older men actually have symptoms of prostate cancer, some cells that seem to have the characteristics of cancer may be present. By the age of 80, a significant number of men will have some cancer in their prostate glands. However, most of these men will never suffer from any symptoms and the cancer may never become a serious threat to health.

Unfortunately, a number of my clients include men went through urological consultations and entered what I call "The Prostate Nightmare". Many of them appeared in my office after aggressive medical treatment (often surgery) for their prostate conditions. While the reason for their treatment (usually a diagnosis of prostate cancer) was no longer an issue, they were suffering from various surgical side effects, such as; erectile dysfunction, inability to orgasm, loss of sensation and others.

And, – it then fell to me to give them the bad news that the medical treatment had damaged, or more likely, destroyed the nerves that were critical for sexual function. I had to explain that my arsenal of herbal and natural treatments would not be effective. Basically, I became the bearer of the bad news that there was no way they would ever recover the natural erectile or orgasm function or sensation they had lost to the treatment.

Many of these men had already accepted the bad news based on their own observations, but needed additional confirmation. Several of them were angry that their doctor did not inform them of the potential for life-long disability prior to their treatment or of alternative treatments that might have saved their functionality. Some of them were mad at me. Most were mad at their doctors. And, some were gratified in the belief that their doctor had saved them from dying of prostate cancer.

As a practitioner that has a strong aversion to alienating my clients, I generally stay away from the fact that they might have had aggressive treatment that was unnecessary, and that their *cancer* might never had been a threat to their life. Recent research has suggested this to be a realistic expectation.

The Numbers Do Not Add Up

The primary method for diagnosing prostate cancer, has, for years been a multiple core needle biopsy. The procedure is usually done by a urologist and guided by an imaging test such as transrectal ultrasound. During the biopsy, the doctor typically takes multiple samples of the prostate using hollow core needles. The tissue in the sample cores is then evaluated by a pathologist.

If the pathologist's report indicated cancer, the man is given a diagnosis of prostate cancer along with a recommendation for immediate treatment, usually surgery. According to the American Cancer Society (ACS), prostate cancer is the most common cancer diagnosed in American men other than skin cancer. They estimate that approximately one-quarter million new cases of prostate cancer (PC) will be diagnosed in 2021 and about 34 thousand men will die of the disease.

According to the ACS, "prostate cancer is the second leading cause of cancer death in American men, behind only lung cancer. About 1 man in 41 will die of prostate cancer."

> These statistics seem to be attached to the top of almost every article I've seen about prostate cancer in the recent past. I suspect many of them are also mentioned to unsuspecting male patients at medical office visits, especially if a prostate cancer diagnosis is on the table. [2]

I challenge these statistics. I have over 1000 male clients in my database. Several hundred have received a diagnosis of prostate cancer. To the best of my knowledge, only one has actually died from prostate cancer in my 20 plus years of practice. This gentlemen had aggressive cancer that spread to his pelvic bones long before it was discovered and he came to me for help.

A medical visit where there is a prostate cancer diagnosis is a visit that is shrouded in apprehension and fear. Often, a man is accompanied by his partner and they are both enveloped in the emotional shock. But, what do these statistics really mean to the shell-shocked patient? Are they just simply misleading, and another way to maximize the impact? Often the patient walks out of the provider's office in shock. In his mind, he is dying from prostate cancer!

Perhaps it is time to analyze and fact check these statistics. Firstly, it takes very little for a man to be given a *prostate cancer* label. However, since this disease is *known* to be deadly, one would expect far more men to actually die from it. The prostate cancer label needs serious qualification.

One of my clients, a 50ish man came to me with a higher than normal PSA result. His doctor was being very cautious with him because his father died of prostate cancer. Further discussion indicated that his father passed away in his late 90's, and that he had several other co-morbidities. He was diagnosed with prostate cancer in his 60's and never received any treatment for it.

I question whether his father actually died of prostate cancer or was it simply a convenient issue. But, I would bet his death was recorded as a prostate cancer statistic. As a layman, I find it kind of strange that a 90 plus man's death is attributed to a condition diagnosed about 35 years earlier.

Now that we have the statistics in place, it seems strange that each of us is not privy to a multitude of friends that have succumbed to prostate cancer. In actuality, the survival rate for PC after diagnosis is over 95 percent. So, how come, each of us that have survived beyond 70, do not have a bevy of friends and relatives that have succumbed to prostate cancer?

Incidentally, that "50ish" client that came to me 20 plus years ago, is still my client, still has an elevated PSA, and is still doing well with no indication of prostate cancer. A 2008 study found that the percentage of prostate cancer in men that had passed away for reasons other than related to the prostate was about equivalent (percentage wise) to the man's age at time of demise.[3]

Many of the autopsies examined at the time of this study, showed an indolent type of prostate cancer. But, almost every man diagnosed with prostate cancer was still referred for aggressive treatment, typically surgery. One of the conclusions of the study authors is posted below:

> "Clinically significant disease should be distinguished from insignificant disease which may pose little or no biological danger to the patient."

The situation is not much different today. The only real difference is that men and their partners are asking more questions and taking more time before they agree to radical surgery to remove their prostates.

However, the doctors giving the diagnosis often do not differentiate between insignificant disease and disease which may become life-threatening. Thus, the poor patient is left to navigate a complex world that he knows little about without a professional guide!

I estimate that a least 10 percent of the clients in my practice were diagnosed with prostate cancer or otherwise told to have their prostates surgically removed. I have confirmed only one death actually attributable to prostate cancer from my group of clients. Many of them have had their prostates removed surgically. All of the men that have had either surgery or radiation are suffering from serious treatment side effects.

The fellow who passed had originally contacted me because he had a PSA test result of more than 50. I advised him to get a repeat PSA in two weeks and call me. Two weeks later he called saying his PSA was now a little over 100. I advised him there was little I could do for him and referred him to a urological specialist I knew in his area as well as the Prostate Cancer Research Organization (PCRI.org). He was diagnosed with metastatic prostate cancer that had spread to his pelvic bones. Six months later, I was advised by a relative that he had passed away.

The purpose of this story is twofold. First – to acknowledge that prostate cancer can indeed be a life-threatening disease, and second to bring to the surface that the threat of dying from it is quite low. In my database for example, the fellow mentioned above is the only one I have knowledge of passing from prostate cancer.

The ACS figures above quote only the total number of cases per year verses the total number of deaths per year. I am not the best mathematician in the world, but a quick calculation on their numbers seems to indicate a death rate of nearly 14 percent.

Considering that the survival rate for prostate cancer posted by experts that treat it daily is better than 95 percent, this indicates, at least to me, that these numbers posted in most of these articles, are, at best, misleading. A cancer diagnosis, even one considered low-risk, can change one's definition of self and can trigger anxiety.

In past 30 or so years, many prostate lesions that were called *cancer* had some cancer characteristics. Cancer has specific characteristics. One of the most important is that its cells tend to spread *uncontrollably*. Today, this fact is indisputable. When one considers patients diagnosed with low-grade cancer (See *Gleason 6 cancer* below*)*, that have not had aggressive treatment, and are not having serious issues with their *cancer* the statistics start to make little sense.

Unfortunately, many practitioners treating men have not yet accepted this finding. And, the unfortunate patients they have treated have experienced massive psychological and physical harm and costs without any clear benefits achieved by their treatment.

The reasons for this are not totally clear, but many are coming to the belief that, since most professionals that treat prostate cancer are urologists and also trained as surgeons, they may be biased towards surgery. However, total removal of the prostate gland is usually unnecessary, and has known, irreversible side effects of incontinence and sexual dysfunction.

The Annual Physical Examination

Just about every man worries about getting prostate cancer. Some worry continuously and their worry can rise to the level of a phobia. For such men, anxiety levels rise as the date of the annual routine physical exam approaches. Their fear makes them very vulnerable to an unscrupulous practitioner.

The annual physical provided by most general practitioners combines a Digital Rectal Examination (DRE) of the prostate along with various routine blood tests, including one for Prostate Specific Antigen (PSA). This is where a prostate nightmare can start. If the doctor detects any abnormality in either the DRE or the PSA test, the patient is usually referred to a urologist for further testing and examination. For years, prostate screening has included the PSA test routinely in many doctors offices, even though it is very non-specific.

The Digital Rectal Examination (DRE) is a routine medical examination typically performed in a general practitioners office. The doctor lubricates a gloved finger and inserts it into the man's rectum. Since the prostate is in close proximity to the rectum, the doctor can feel much of the prostate surface through the rectal passage. If the prostate surface is not smooth or has irregularities such as lumps, the DRE is said to be suspicious. This often results in a prostate biopsy.

One of my clients came to me after his urologist recommended he have a prostate biopsy after a lump was found on his prostate during the routine DRE. He had already gone through eight prostate biopsies during the past few years, each ordered by the same urologist and initiated by the same DRE finding. Each of these biopsies was negative for cancer.

Common sense would dictate that this man had a lump on his prostate that was likely a benign structural deformity unique to him. However, each year, he was subjected to a biopsy that caused him significant pain and bleeding as well as some erectile dysfunction for more than a month. Even though multiple biopsies had been performed over several years, and, my client had no symptoms whatsoever, his doctor was still recommending another biopsy.

Part of the medical paradigm is to isolate and treat disease – but this does not always allow for a common sense approach. Another part of the medical doctrine is *primum non nocere* – which in Latin means – "First, do no harm."

Biopsy needles do harm to the prostate! Perhaps the damage is minimal, but it is damage and the long-term effects of multiple biopsies have not, to the best of my knowledge, ever been seriously studied.

This particular patient had been subjected to the harms of a biopsy several times for no real purpose, except possibly the urologist was covering his tracks in case cancer showed up later in this patient. The physician could always use the legal defense that he did everything any of his peers would do in a similar circumstance – a valid legal defense. Unfortunately, providing a doctor the legal means to avoid a future lawsuit is not always conducive to the well-being of the patient!

However, to the patient, if a doctor is hinting that he may have prostate cancer, worry can take precedence over common sense, especially if the provider is quoting death from prostate cancer statistics.

The PSA Test

Prostate Specific Antagen (PSA) screening was introduced in the US around 1987 and approved by the FDA as a prostate cancer screening tool around 1994. PSA is a substance produced only by the male prostate gland. It tends to increase with age as well as when the prostate has some kind of problem.

Testing caught on rapidly in the US, and the number of men over 50 diagnosed with prostate cancer has skyrocketed since. This begs the question of whether or not such intense screening for prostate cancer actually saves lives or causes more problems. Since the advent of PSA testing to routine blood work for men over fifty, the rate of men diagnosed with prostate cancer has increased substantially.

The PSA blood test is typically performed by a man's regular doctor during a routine annual blood draw. PSA is produced by the male prostate gland and can become elevated as a result of any change in the environment around the prostate. Typical causes for an elevated PSA can be recent sexual activity, infection, bicycle or motorcycle riding, gland enlargement (BPH), as well as prostate cancer.

Unfortunately, many men get information and advice about tests like the PSA from friends on the golf course and/or gym. Often, the advice of his peers is somber when a man discloses his PSA is above normal. This alone is a psychological motivation for more treatment and fear.

However, an elevated PSA can have multiple causes and it is, at best, a very poor indicator of possible cancer. Over more than twenty years of practice, I have met many men with elevated PSA readings. For the vast majority of them, it was a temporary rise due to some kind of transient activity or condition and dropped on a subsequent test.

Some of my long-term clients have had a slowly rising PSA value over about the past ten years. This out-of-range PSA usually results in a prostate biopsy being ordered. However, each of these clients refused the biopsy and seem to be physically well, although one of them is approaching the age of 95.

One measurement, called PSA density, takes into account prostate enlargement in the resulting PSA value. For a man, like myself, that has severe BPH, this calculation allows for higher values of PSA to be considered before recommending a biopsy. My slowly rising PSA began more than 20 years ago, and I have yet to have any treatment aside from dietary changes, some herbal supplements and exercise.

However, many doctors do not consider PSA density as a viable measure. Most also order biopsies. The reason for this could be a measure of thoroughness as well as simply greed. A biopsy generates more revenue.

The men that I met were the lucky ones. Many balked at the prospect of having more medical tests and/or procedures based on the outcome of their single out-of-range PSA test and sought guidance from an independent medical source or a natural health practitioner.

Other men accepted the advice given to them by the doctor they were visiting at the time. Usually, most of them went on to aggressive treatment that was likely unnecessary, and thus, they entered the area I call the *prostate nightmare* – a diagnosis of prostate cancer and subsequent aggressive treatment.

Such a diagnosis can result in extreme duress and is often coupled in many men (as well as their partners) with an emotional need for immediate treatment to “fix” or “remove” the problem. But since most “cancers” found via routine PSA testing are clinically insignificant, aggressive treatment can be much more damaging than helpful—especially to a man's quality of life as well as his sexual relationship.

> Men diagnosed with prostate cancer are frequently scheduled for aggressive treatment shortly after their diagnosis. Much of this is due to misinformation on the part of the patient, and a failure of the clinician to fully explain the risk/benefit ratio. It is often easier to satisfy an emotional need of a patient for immediate treatment, than it is to explain to a panicky patient and his partner that his cancer may never become life threatening. [4]

This results in the well-known over-treatment of many cases of localized, low-risk, non-aggressive lesions inadvertently diagnosed as prostate cancer. The diagnosis of low-risk, non-aggressive cancer is typically the bulk of patients being treated currently. Unfortunately, all prostate cancer treatment has significant side effects, particularly on a man's quality of life.

Without question, all treatment for prostate cancer – short of watchful waiting – causes some degree of permanent sexual or urinary dysfunction. While some function may return after a few weeks or months, **it will never be the same as it was before treatment.** Many men go into treatment without fully understanding this—only to regret it later. To put this simply, some urinary incontinence may self-resolve in time. So, after a while you may be able to urinate close to normally. However, sexual function, even if it resolves to the point of being able to get an erection, will *never* be the same.

In today's society, we are conditioned to quickly treat all health problems that occur. Couple this mindset with the word *cancer*, and panic can easily set in. A doctor that feels immediate treatment is not mandatory may well find himself transferring patient records to someone else—even though a man with low-risk prostate cancer may be well advised to pursue a program of "watchful-waiting" or "active surveillance"—especially if he is 75 or older.

For many men and their clinicians though, "watchful waiting" simply means a repeat PSA test and biopsy every few months. During this time, if cancer is actually present, the original conditions that caused it to appear are not altered, and thus one is only waiting for the cancer to progress to a point where aggressive medical treatment is mandatory. Meanwhile, the repeat biopsies are doing structural damage to the working prostate.

Prostate Biopsy

A prostate biopsy is typically ordered almost as a reflex action to an elevated PSA result, even if a DRE is totally unremarkable. There are several reasons for this; First, many urologists simply believe it is in the best interest of the patient; Second, if a biopsy is not done and a serious cancer later ensues, the urologist may be facing related legal issues.

> This begs the question, – Is this in the best interest of the patient? In most cases, the answer is an unqualified NO! A biopsy is an aggressive procedure that can carry a bunch of complications as well as leading the way to more complicated and unneeded procedures. The only purpose of a biopsy is to determine if prostate cancer is present, AND serious enough to need treatment. If there is little likelihood of a serious condition, the biopsy serves little function.[5]
>
> ***Regardless of what your doctor tells you, post-procedure complications from prostate biopsies are common, can be quite serious, and, in some cases, life-threatening!***

One study reported approximately 40 percent of the men experienced a complication from a biopsy, and the rate of complications rose to nearly 60 percent for men that had 24 core samples taken instead of a lower sample rate.

The most common complication is a post-procedure infection. Keep in mind that a prostate biopsy is done with a probe inserted through the rectum for access to the prostate. Men are typically given a chemical enema (known as a Fleet enema) prior to the procedure, to lower the amount of fecal material in the rectum prior to inserting the biopsy probe. However, no matter how strong or efficient the enema is, some E. Coli bacteria will still be present in the rectum and some of it will inevitably be carried into the prostate as the procedure is performed.

A biopsy induced infection is almost always due to fecal matter driven into the prostate by the biopsy needles as they pass through the rectum. This kind of infection can be relatively benign or severe enough to lead to hospitalization, prolonged antibiotic therapy, and secondary adverse events.

Several years ago, I was in the position of being told that I needed a prostate biopsy. My urologist at the time told me there was "absolutely no risk" of infection. Questioning that, I was firmly assured it was true, as he handed me a prescription for a powerful antibiotic to start taking the day before the procedure. When I questioned him about this, he looked at me as if I had six heads. (I never went back to him.)

A few weeks after my encounter, the wife of one of my friends (also a patient of this same doctor), called me to tell me that her husband was in the hospital with a prostate biopsy induced infection. He survived, but, ...

Experts estimate that about a million prostate biopsy procedures are performed each year in the United States. Some are used to monitor known cancers, but the majority are for diagnosis of possible new cases. The procedure has been used for many years as the "gold standard" for diagnosis of prostate cancer. While prostate cancer is a very common diagnosis, especially the Gleason 6 kind (explained below) it is life-threatening in only a relatively few men.

However, there are numerous other ways to diagnose prostate cancer that do not involve an aggressive biopsy. It is way beyond the scope of this book to enumerate the multiple ways prostate cancer can be diagnosed without a biopsy. However, I suggest any man considering further examination of his prostate for cancer, familiarize himself with all available options.

A report from Oregon Health & Science University published in 2005 detailed several different techniques for diagnosing prostate cancer without a biopsy. This report, was summarized and published in Science Daily. Although is nearly 25 years old, it is still pertinent.

Implementation of a Prostate Biopsy

A prostate biopsy is a procedure whose aim is to identify prostate cancer. During the procedure a tool containing multiple hollow sample needles is inserted into the rectum. This tool may also contain a camera or ultrasonic probe as a guide. Its intended purpose is to stab a hollow needle into the prostate and extract that needle with a portion of prostate tissue in it. The ultimate goal is to take multiple samples from different areas and pass the prostate tissue from the hollow needles along to a pathologist for examination. Thus, the more tissue extracted the higher the possibility of finding an abnormality – and the greater the damage done to the prostate.

It is best to keep in mind the logistics of a prostate biopsy. Generally, older men have a prostate that is be larger than the textbook walnut size. I have met men whose prostate is about the size of a peach. Note that the size of the prostate is not an indicator of whether or not it is diseased. An enlarged prostate has not been implicated to affect the risk of developing prostate cancer. Most older men have a condition called BPH or Benign Prostate Enlargement. BPH is not linked to cancer and does not increase the risk of getting prostate cancer. By its very nature, a large prostate dictates that more core tissue samples be taken, increasing the trauma to the prostate.

Secondly, from the viewpoint of a urologist. Biopsy equipment cost can unconsciously factor into a decision of whether or not to biopsy or how many biopsies to perform. While this should not be the case, human nature being what it is, it most certainly can be a factor. A quick search at the time of this writing found that a complete prostate biopsy setup was for sale on Ebay for about $70,000. Thus, a practice that does a lot of biopsies can generate a larger profit from the equipment quicker.

The cost of a prostate biopsy to the patient was estimated at about $2000 in 2020. However, any complications can drive the cost up substantially. A single complication, like an infection, can easily double the cost, while a complication requiring hospitalization can drive it into the middle to high figures. In most cases, insurance pays the cost.

From the urologists point of view, about 30 or so uncomplicated biopsies need to be performed to recover the basic costs of the machine. This, of course, does not cover the salaries of the support personnel involved in performing and/or following up on patients. The bottom line is that a prostate biopsy can easily result in a five figure bill to the patient. If a patient has minimal or no health insurance, there can be substantial cost..

Considering that, even with a 24 core biopsy, there is still a possibility that all of the biopsy needles might miss an area containing cancerous tissue in a large prostate. Obviously this renders the particular biopsy useless.

To diagnose cancer, one or more of the core samples in a biopsy has to pass into or through an area of the prostate that contains abnormal tissue. Thus, the more core samples taken, the higher the likelihood of passing into or through abnormal tissue. The obvious goal is to pass a narrow needle through diseased tissue to take a sample. But considering the fact that the diseased tissue may simply be a limited to a small area, it is quite possible that the biopsy needles go right by a suspicious area without sampling it.

Most biopsies are done using ultrasound to guide the probe and needles to areas that look suspicious. However, there is no guarantee that this is effective. Thus, even if a prostate biopsy does not show any abnormality, prostate cancer may still be present.

Thus, begins one part of what I call the *prostate nightmare* – While in some cases, the test is accurate, there is always some uncertainty. – Is cancer present, or not?

The other side of this coin is that the pathologist examining the tissue removed during the biopsy does not want to make a mistake. Pathologists are human, and they know that an error might mean a matter of life or death. An honest error on the conservative side might make the difference between saving a life or dooming a man to unnecessary life-long side effects and complications.

There is considerable controversy among professionals working in the prostate cancer realm as to the definition of prostate cancer. The common diagnosis of Gleason 6 prostate cancer is under question as to whether it actually is cancer or not.

The definition of cancer includes *uncontrolled cell growth.* It is hard to apply this definition to a condition that might be in a man's body for years without causing any severe problems.

The Typical "Gleason 6" Biopsy Result

According to the American Cancer Institute statistics, more then 250,000 men receive a prostate cancer label yearly. However, since the survival rate is typically greater than 95 percent, it seems this is a strong indicator that prostate cancer is not the a serious, potentially fatal disease requiring immediate surgical treatment that many urological specialists deem it to be.

Basically, there are two types of prostate cancer:

• A very common form, often called indolent prostate cancer. It is the kind that presents as a small localized tumor in the prostate that remains relatively small and is very slow-growing. This is the kind of tissue that is represented in the vast majority of diagnosed prostate cancers. It is generally not life-threatening and men can often live with it for many, many years. It is often characterized as "Gleason 6 cancer," referencing the cancer grade as described by Dr. Donald Gleason in the 1960s. This classification, defined over 60 years ago, is the yardstick still used today. The most common presentation is a Gleason 6 score. Many experts question if this should be considered cancer or not. Unfortunately, nearly every man diagnosed with Gleason 6 prostate cancer today is subjected to aggressive treatment.

• A less common form, representing less than 10 percent of the lesions found, is rated higher than Gleason 6, with Gleason scoes of 7 through 10. This smaller percentage is a real cancer which can be aggressive and might be likely to metastasize and thus needs attention and treatment.

Understanding the significance of the *cancer* label is very important since it is an established fact that most men given the *prostate cancer* label will be aggressively treated, most often with surgery. And, if their cancer is of a type that is insignificant, non-killer indolent variety, the treatment will commonly leave them with debilitating treatment after-effects and zero benefit.

The "cancer" label is typically qualified by the Gleason grading score. This score attempts to determine the significance of a particular "cancer" by estimating the amount of what appears to be cancerous tissue in each of the cores removed in a biopsy. In most cases, insignificant cancer is given a Gleason score of 6, and, depending on the point of view of the urologist, often treated the same as an aggressive cancer, with a recommendation of surgery.

This method of using the "Gleason" score to classify prostate cancer is a very established practice that has been used for years. However, considering that this Gleason 6 "cancer" may not really cancer at all, diagnosis and overtreatment is common. In essence, this is nothing more than exploitation of vulnerable men and their partners by the prostate cancer industry. For many years, it has resulted in significant overtreatment and surgical harm to patients.

> While the Gleason 6 score is quite common and generally insignificant, any man receiving a Gleason score of 7 or higher needs to take the diagnosis seriously and investigate all his options for treatment. But, painting of the Gleason 6 grade with the same brush as a "must treat" cancer, as many urologists tend to do, is at best misleading, and at worst borders on exploitation for profit. **Only 10 to 15 percent of prostate cancers with significant amounts of Gleason 4 or 5 are considered high-risk and are potentially deadly without treatment.** [6]

Recently, several well-known experts in the prostate cancer field have published articles and books concerning prostate cancer screening, management and/or treatment. These doctors have the fortitude to challenge the conventional prostate cancer wisdom. Unfortunately, their voices are often lost in the cacophony of *conventional wisdom.*

Many professions have high inertia when it comes to new ideas, even when the new ideas come from highly respected members of the community. On the last page of my book "*Your Prostate, Your Libido, Your Life*" I relate the case of Dr. Ignaz Philipp Semmelweis. I have quoted what I said in that book below;

> *In medicine, this inertia can result in inadvertent harm to its patients. In the mid 19th century, Hungarian physician Ignaz Philipp Semmelweis was abused, criticized, and ostracized for his promotion of the idea that doctors should wash their hands after delivering an infant. He suggested that the death of many mothers due to fevers after childbirth was caused by the failure of physicians to wash their hands between deliveries. It was more than two decades before his ideas were even partially accepted—even though he significantly reduced the incidence of both mother and infant mortality by implementing this procedure in his clinics. Today, Semmelweis is considered to be one of the great physicians of his time."*

Unfortunately, cases like this still abound. About the middle of the last century, Dr. Linus Pauling postulated that intravenous Vitamin C might be able to cure cancer and help many other conditions. He was also ridiculed for his statements. In 2020, many nursing homes began using his findings to help alleviate suffering from Covid-19. However, very little research has yet to be published.

The study referenced below sparked controversy simply because it recognized that there is a common early stage lesion found in the prostate that has, until now, been classified and treated as if it were a potentially aggressive cancer. These lesions do not have the clinical course that would likely evolve into life-threatening disease. The result was that guidelines were issued that emphasized the need for more informed discussions between patients and clinicians prior to treatment intervention. However, the guidelines do not specify that clinicians honestly convey treatment-associated adverse effect information to their patients.

> Thus, the common Gleason 6 prostate cancer diagnosis may not be cancer at all. But, once this label has been attached to a patient's record, every doctor and nurse associated with treating the patient is essentially on alert for more cancer. Unfortunately, some doctors do not recognize the harm this mindset is putting patients through. [7]

When prostate samples are examined under a microscope, a pathologist in the laboratory looks to see how closely the cells resemble those of normal tissue. The samples are rated on a scale of 3 (most similar to healthy tissue) to 5 (least similar), then the two most common grades together to determine what's called the Gleason score. The most common Gleason 6 score results when the two common grades are both 3.

Gleason 6 is the lowest possible grade. This rating means that the prostate cancer is considered to be low- or very low-risk disease. Most of these tumors are found during routine prostate cancer screenings.

Gleason 6 prostate tumors grow slowly and may never cause a problem – or even need treatment. Progressive urologists realize this and guide their patients towards active surveillance rather than immediate surgery.

What Exactly is "The Prostate Nightmare?"

Our society has morphed "cancer" into a very frightening word. The threat of any kind of cancer strikes fear in many people. Prostate cancer generates uncertainty and *fear* in virtually all men and their partners. Every guy has heard stories about a colleague that had prostate cancer, and, as a result is living with a completely destroyed sex life, urinary incontinence and other symptoms. And, this poor quality life will likely remain for the remainder of his life.

Many of my clients have related the story of their cancer diagnosis. A typical scenario, summarized from several patient stories goes as follows:

> "My wife and I were very anxious to hear about the results of my prostate biopsy initiated after my PSA score was deemed higher than it should be. I was also anxious about when the biopsy side effects I was suffering would subside. Doctor X walked into the office where his nurse had directed us, and sat down behind his desk. He was shuffling through a folder, which I assumed was mine. After a minute or two, he announced calmly, 'Well, Mr. Y, it appears you have prostate cancer. We need to get you on the schedule for surgery immediately.' He looked up, nonchalantly raised his reading glasses, and asked if we had any questions."

This scenario is all too common. Even if the patient or his partner did have questions, they were likely stymied by the huge mental shock of the matter-of-fact diagnosis they had just received.

This is what I call "the prostate nightmare." It strikes many men. Starting with a visit to their doctor for their annual physical when they are found to have either an abnormal DRE or an abnormal PSA. This sets in motion a series of events that are almost exclusively controlled by the man's doctors and corresponding urological medical practice.

It is a rare man indeed that can stand firm in the face of a somber-faced medical practitioner telling him that he is taking a huge chance with his life by not agreeing to have an immediate prostate biopsy or surgery. It is very rare for a doctor to explain the drawbacks and side effects of these procedures.

Here are some real case studies that are (unfortunately) quite common;

- **Case 1** – A 52 YO man, in generally good health and reasonably fit physically, woke up at about 3 am on a Sunday morning, and was totally unable to urinate. By late morning, he was taken by his two sons to the local ER, where, after allowing him to suffer until early afternoon, a nurse finally catheterized him, emptying more than a liter of urine from his painful bladder.

  By late afternoon, a urologist visited with him and he was told, in no uncertain terms, that he needed surgery to remove his prostate. He was told the surgery was routine and they could schedule it first thing in the morning. He would be in the hospital for a few days and would be able to return to work within about a week.

  There was virtually no discussion about side effects of the surgery or life after prostate removal. Just that the procedure was routine and life would be back to normal within a short time.

The surgery was performed on a Monday morning and the patient returned to his hospital room by mid-afternoon for recovery. The recovery proceeded until the mid-evening when a blood clot broke loose from the surgical area. The man suffered a pulmonary thrombosis and expired shortly thereafter.

Summary – The year was 1963. The man in question was my 52 YO father. He suffered from BPH, but back in 1963 in the US, a prostatectomy was considered the gold standard of treatment for most prostate issues, including BPH. In Europe at the time, they were successfully using herbals like saw palmetto and flower pollen as first line treatment for BPH.

- **Case 2** – An 86 YO man, having intermittent difficulty urinating on his own, visits a urologist and gets a recommendation for a Transurethral Prostatectomy (TURP). His nephew, a client of mine, called for my opinion, and, after hearing about the man's other co-morbidities, I recommended he find another way to resolve the problem.

My suggestion was that he learn to use self-cathetherization when he cannot urinate on his own. Considering that the man's other morbidities required nursing assistance and his wife was a permanent caretaker with nursing experience, this appeared to be a reasonable approach.

However, at the insistence of the practitioner, the man was convinced to have the procedure. He expired about 30 days later from complications of the surgery and his co-morbidities.

- **Case 3** – A 65 YO man, presented in the ER in severe discomfort due to his inability to empty his bladder from the night before. This patient was morbidly obese and had been having urinary symptoms for several days. After catheterizing him, he was released to a urological practice that immediately scheduled him for a prostate biopsy.

> I suggested he see an out of town urologist that I knew personally. After examining him and performing a color-Doppler scan of his prostate, the urologist diagnosed a urinary/prostate infection (prostatitis) and prescribed an antibiotic to treat it.
>
> Within a few days, his immediate urinary problem subsided. I advised him that without addressing his weight and overall health, he was heading down a path towards some kind of disaster – urinary or otherwise. But, a few months later, he had the same problem again, and went back to his original urologist who convinced him to have his prostate surgically removed.
>
> The next time I heard from him was about two years later when he came to me to in an attempt to recover his sexual function. He had not had an erection since the surgery and everything his doctor had tried did not work. He was devastated when I told him there was little I could do to help him.

I could extract many more examples from my files, but the above three seem to summarize the main points. Men have little to no knowledge of the overall function of their prostate glands, and, when there is dysfunction, they suspend their intelligence in deference to someone with perceived higher knowledge. Most often, this person is a urologist, and it most often results in aggressive treatment that they really do not need.

Fear of the dreaded prostate cancer diagnosis combined with an over zealous practitioner can easily send a man down a path of medical tests and procedures that may permanently alter his quality of life.

The watchword for the *prostate nightmare* is *fear*. The practitioner is stoking the man's and his partner's fear. It really doesn't, matter if is a conscious or subconscious stoking. The fear of prostate cancer is real, whether or not that fear is justified or not, it is a strong motivator for the man to agree to additional diagnostic testing and/or procedures. A stone-faced doctor confirming that his fear is real, will usually convince the man and his wife to accept the recommendations and go along with the recommendation.

The end result is that, if the routine tests show any discrepancy from what the practitioner considers normal, additional tests and procedures will most certainly be ordered. And, aggressive treatment will often be initiated.

Surgeons are well aware that the *cancer* word generates considerable anxiety, disbelief and a desperate turn towards "survival mode" for many patients and their partners. Unfortunately, time and again, physicians egos and greed cloud their ability to recognize and change bad treatment philosophies. Physicians that steadfastly adhere to harmful or outdated protocols are often the biggest obstacles to intelligent medical progress.

With older men and prostate issues, this resistance to change, along with a cookie-cutter approach by many urologists has perpetuated male misery for many years.

> The "*Prostate Cancer Nightmare*" is a condition that befalls an unwary man and his partner. Somehow, the medical diagnosis, correct or incorrect, induces an ability for them to short-circuit and suspend their intellect due to fear of succumbing to prostate cancer. This leaves them very

vulnerable to suggestions that death will occur if the recommended treatment plan is not followed. In most cases, the only death that occurs is to the man's quality of life! [8]

The Cookie Cutter Approach

Many doctors, particularly urologists, use a "cookie cutter" approach to diagnosing and treating their patients. Each patient gets basically the same treatment, regardless of the reason for the initial consult. One of my clients provided a good example of this approach as he related the story of his visit to a urologist.

After his consult with the doctor, he received a phone call at home from the doctor's scheduler, who told him the doctor had ordered a prostate biopsy for him. This particular client had gone to several consults with this doctor before and had made it known to the doctor that he had been diagnosed with rectal cancer a couple years before.

The cancer diagnosis had led him to have part of his colon as well as his entire rectum removed surgically. He now had an colostomy taking the place of his normal rectal stool passageway. His entire rectal passage as well as the anal opening had been removed surgically and replaced by an ostomy pouch on his lower abdomen. The procedure he had was called an abdomino-perineal-resection or APR.

It is a procedure that results in part of the colon relocated to the abdomen where it is brought through the abdominal wall and serves as the opening for the removal of stool. It is also a procedure that surgically removes the anal opening and rectum.

The abdominal opening is formed by drawing the part of the colon through an incision in the anterior abdominal wall and suturing it into place. This opening is typically used in conjunction with a removable pouch to collect the stool. It provides an alternative channel for feces to be removed from the body when the rectum and anus are no longer functional.

Since the rectum is no longer used, it is typically removed as a part of the surgery. The anal sphincter muscle that surrounds the rectal opening is removed as well leaving the patient to expel stool from the ostomy for the rest of his life.

So, since the physician had this noted in his records, is should have been obvious that a prostate biopsy through the rectum was not possible for this patient. I could chalk this up to a simple mistake except that my client had made the scheduler aware of the situation when she attempted to schedule his appointment. Nonetheless, she said she would talk to the doctor about it and get back to the patient.

He received a call the next day telling him the doctor insisted that he needed the biopsy and he should schedule it. There is only one reason for this disaster; the doctor's employees had been pre-trained to eliminate all patient presented obstacles to the doctor's performance of a biopsy, even if the obstacle resulted in making the procedure (as planned by the urologist), totally impossible physically. This is a gross example of the cookie-cutter approach used by some unethical urologists.

The office staff had been trained to fend off any attempts by a patient to avoid the "cookie cutter" approach to a procedure. In my opinion, perhaps the patient should have made the appointment and kept it. Imagine the surprise of the doctor and staff as they tried to insert the biopsy probe into the patients non-existent rectum.

The Emotional Impact of a Prostate Cancer Diagnosis

A few years ago I was associated with a website for men that had prostate cancer. We put out a survey to get a feeling for how treated men reacted emotionally and physically post treatment. The level of regret was about the same for a radical prostatectomy or radiation therapy. Men that had chosen active surveillance were less regretful.

The single biggest contributor to regret was treatment-associated sexual dysfunction, seconded only by regret that they had agreed to treatment without a full understanding of the ramifications. Most of the men had serious regrets about not knowing the sexual side effects would be so severe.

Many said they were aware that erectile dysfunction might be a side effect. To them, erectile dysfunction was something they had dealt with before and could live with. However, many of them were not aware that the erectile dysfunction as a result of treatment would be so all encompassing. One guy told me, "It is like I'm dead down there. I get aroused mentally, but feel nothing physically."

Men who have low-risk disease and choose active surveillance can avoid treatment-associated harms like incontinence and impotence, but they still have the severe impact of the diagnosis itself. A diagnosis of prostate cancer is devastating, even if it is wrong!

A survey of almost 1,000 patients showed that the diagnosis itself is debilitating. I met with some patients whose only concern prior to treatment was to remove the cancer, regardless of the consequences. As a group, these men were more accepting of their treatment-induced side effects, but also expressed thoughts that they should have done more research prior to treatment.

Clinical practice could be significantly improved to ensure men are adequately informed of the potential consequences. Many doctors routinely screen older men without considering the fact that some of them may not want to consider screening. Many men expressed the view that their doctor did not accurately inform them of the potential side effects of screening or treatment.

> A recent report concluded that after several years of introspection, about 15 percent of men with localized prostate cancer regretted the decisions they made regarding treatment. I suspect this report is very biased. Based on my own informal study, I believe the real number is likely several times higher. [9]

Within my own practice, more than half the men I interviewed who had treatment in the form of surgery or radiation were regretful of their treatment decision. The mental health side effects of treatment were worse among men that were highly sexually motivated prior to the treatment. Most had issues with self-esteem and all of them rated their current sexual experiences as much less rewarding than prior to their treatment.

For a short period of time a few years ago, I served as the coodinator of a local Red Cross sponsored support group for men with prostate cancer. Most of the men came to the group to share their treatment stories with peers that were in a similar situation. Throughout my tenure as coordinator, I never met a anyone who openly expressed regret about his treatment decision. However, I did meet several wives that were more candid.

Psychologically, it is hard for many of us to admit minor mistakes, so I can sympathize with how hard it is for a guy to admit he made his treatment decision exclusively on the recommendation of his doctor. This seems to be especially true when he is surrounded by other men in a peer group. Imagine how difficult it is for a man to admit he made the wrong decision, especially if he is suffering severe treatment-related sexual inadequacy.

To folks that study human psychology, this fits into cognitive dissonance theory. By assigning a positive value to the outcome, they can accept that their decision was justified. In other words, "I am now free of prostate cancer" justifies they made the right decision – in their mind.

The problem with this is that there is a strong possibility that they were over-diagnosed and did not really have prostate cancer to begin with.

The Truth About Prostate Cancer

Contrary to the generally accepted myths propagated by the media and others, most men diagnosed with prostate cancer do not die from it. Prostate cancer can be a serious disease, but there is no evidence that men diagnosed and treated for it actually live longer or have a better quality of life than men that receive no treatment. If fact, – It seems the opposite may is true.

The major problem is that the medical paradigm for diagnosing prostate cancer has been in place with little change for close to 30 years. Considering our litigious social environment, many of the clinicians that normally diagnose diseases like prostate cancer are cautious. They are always aware of the litigious environment they have been thrust into, and are thus, often overzealous in making a diagnosis.

The result is that virtually any anomaly in the prostate is likely to receive a prostate cancer diagnosis. Thus, the prostate cancer label can easily be applied to almost all lesions whether or not they are significant.

This all-inclusive label sets the bar for multiple additional diagnostic tests as well as "*curative*" surgery. It is blatantly deceptive. Men are told they have prostate cancer, and, with their partners, suffer the grief, dismay and emotional distress of this serious, life-threatening diagnosis. Thus, this diagnosis, often with no real scientific justification, is locked into patient's medical record and follows him to every clinician he subsequently consults with.

Psychologically, when a cancer label is applied by a physician, many men, along with their partners go through a series of emotions. Denial and doubt is first, followed by disbelief, and finally acceptance. Often, very intelligent patients suspend their intelligence and accept their clinicians recommendations. Others, go through a stage of researching various treatments for their *cancer* in the hope of finding a treatment that is less debilitating and has fewer side effects.

There are many treatments for prostate cancer. There are also many treatments that are used for men that have been diagnosed with prostate cancer, but unaware that their diagnosis is incorrect. Most of them have their prostates surgically removed or irradiated and then suffer the side effects of the treatment for the rest of their life.

Being involved with older men with prostate issues for many years has taught me that there is little to gain by telling a man that who had his prostate surgically removed that there is no hope for recovering sexual function.

Disability from surgical trauma and destruction to the internal erection controlling nerves is not conducive to repair. The best outcome is usually that he now accepts his loss. A typical response is "Well, at least my doc cut the prostate cancer out of me." or, "I don't have prostate cancer anymore."

For many of these men, my answer could easily be "You probably never really had prostate cancer," but, aside from that bordering on a path to cruelty, it also guarantees a complete loss of credibility with my client! Often, people believe what they have been told simply because it is too painful to admit the truth.

A few years ago, I was involved with a prostate health site that put out a survey asking their members (almost exclusively prostatectomy patients) if they would undergo the same treatment for their "prostate cancer" again. More that 90 percent responded that they would. When the members were further questioned, the almost universal response was that, "they were now cancer-free." This begs the question of "what if you did not really have cancer?"

This is a cultural issue, not a medical one! For decades, the conventional medical community has been promoting the idea that cancer is potentially curable when it is detected early. While this is likely true of many cancers, it has no basis for a diagnosis of cancer that is incorrect!

Many of the men in the survey quoted above probably did not have prostate cancer. Yet, they were treated for it. And, more that 90 percent of them are happy with the treatment because, "they are now cancer-free." They have emotionally accepted the outcome because to admit that it was an error is simply too painful.

And, topping this off, statistics indicate the survival rate for men after a prostate cancer diagnoses is well over 90 percent. This begs the question of whether or not we are actually treating a deadly disease, or putting a man through an extensive life-altering event such as prostate surgery that is actually doing nothing to prevent his untimely demise and may even be hastening it!

For a man and his partner, enveloped in fear and wholly convinced that his prostate cancer will kill him, the prospect of having his prostate and the cancer within it totally removed, is very enticing, even if it has some side effects. I have had many of my clients relate the conversation between themselves and their practitioner where the implied scenario was that the prostate cancer would kill him if he did not have the recommended treatment.

The fact is that many men that actually do have low-risk prostate cancer live with it for many years. My paternal uncle was diagnosed with prostate cancer at about 60 YO. Due to his older brother's (my father) untimely death from prostate surgery, he was strongly out of tune with his urological recommendation. He lived until his late 80's and died from a stroke while he still had prostate cancer.

What is Cancer?

According to most experts. Cancer refers to any one of a large number of diseases characterized by the development of abnormal cells that divide uncontrollably. Thus, such cells may infiltrate (metastasize) to other places and potentially destroy normal body tissue.

Considering the above definition, it is surprising that several million men that have been diagnosed with prostate cancer at some point in their lives are still alive today.

A good comparison to a prostate cancer for a man is a diagnosis of ductile carcinoma in-sutu or DCIS for a woman. Conventional thinking considers this an early form of breast cancer with a low risk of being invasive. It is usually diagnosed from a mammogram as part of routine breast cancer screening. Like prostate cancer, it does not quite fit the defined rule for cancer, but it is presented to the patient as a cancer needing treatment. Again, like prostate cancer, treatment can be aggressive.

In essence, the only difference between this scenario and the one for prostate cancer is that the patient's gender is different and the somber-faced medical practitioner is typically a gynecologist rather than a urologist. Both patients face the same emotional consequences and distress, with the man facing a decision about removing his prostate and the woman facing surgery that may result in loss of her breasts.

The similarity in both of these scenarios is that a seemingly well patient is devastated by a totally unexpected diagnosis and recommendation for serious treatment that will cause significant disability, – at least for a time.

In today's world the medical establishment controls the diagnosis and treatment of disease. Citizens are bombarded by daily media advertisements for various drugs and treatments. Within each media piece is the *order* to call your doctor to see if this drug is right for you. In advertising this is called the CTA or call to action.

But, what if you actually heed this advice and call or visit your doctor. Will you actually get some specific advice or be thrust into the "cookie cutter" mill again? In today's medical mill environment it is very likely you will encounter the latter.

Consider the following – your car is running poorly. You take it to a mechanic and are told that it needs a new *frammis* that will cost you about $1000. You have the choice of accepting the fix **or** taking your vehicle to another mechanic for a second opinion.

After a prostate or breast cancer diagnosis, you also have a choice to go for a second opinion, but this game is played with differing rules. While the mechanic you choose for a second opinion can be totally independent from the first, your second medical opinion will likely be a practitioner that is either a urologist or a gynecologist. Also, your second opinion doctor will likely be looking at the same scans and data collected by the first practitioner. It is also very possible that he/she will be following the exact same treatment or diagnosis protocols.

Thus, the potential for both practitioners agreeing on the diagnosis is quite high. In other words, you are stuck in a loop with no viable exit except to forgo treatment completely or succumb to the doctor's recommendation.

However, it is rare for a patient and his partner to have the emotional fortitude to stand up to somber-faced medical personnel predicting "doom and gloom" on failure to follow the medical recommendations. Unfortunately, many patients opt for treatment and later regret it.

The Truth About Treatments for Prostate Cancer

There are many treatments being promoted for prostate cancer. In this article we talk mostly about the radical prostatectomy since it is the most common treatment currently used in the US. However, it is not the only treatment and many men diagnosed with Gleason 6 succumb to the belief that they must treat their diagnosed prostate cancer or risk dying. Often, they also may want to research different treatments that may have more tolerable side effects.

Thus, they seek out information of various other types of treatment for their prostate cancer. Their goal at this point is to find a treatment that is tolerable for them. The thought never occurs that the prostate cancer diagnosis might be incorrect or that it may not need treatment. Emotionally, they have accepted their cancer diagnosis and are looking for a way to resolve it that has the least effect on their quality of life.

Unfortunately, regardless of what a practicing doctor might imply, **there is no treatment for prostate cancer that does not have side effects.** Almost all treatments for this condition have the same side effects, albeit at differing levels. A radical prostatectomy has side effects that occur almost immediately after the surgery. Radiation therapy might have side effects that do not appear until months or sometimes years later.

Active surveillance, formerly known as watchful waiting, can often be a very productive arrangement. While it is not a cure, it allows the means to keep watch on a questionable situation to see if there is any negative progress on it. However, this process does not appeal to everyone. Some men feel that it is "doing nothing" and balk at it.

Psychologically, the thought of "doing nothing" is contrary to the mental image conveyed by the current thoughts of today. In our modern world, you treat cancer or die! The medical profession, with few exceptions seems to promote this paradigm. While it may be effective for some cancers, I firmly believe that most diagnoses of prostate cancer are indolent and do not require immediate treatment.

I have been recommending watchful waiting for some of my clients for more than 20 years. To date, only one client has seen a progression in his condition that required additional treatment. The others have gone along with their lives with few problems that could be attributed to their prostate.

Unfortunately though, the conventional medical mindset has been drilled into everyone. Both the medical establishment and media are guilty of this. Many people believe that the best way to get rid of cancer is to "cut it out!" While this may be true of certain fast-growing aggressive cancers, it has certainly been disproved for most prostate cancer.

Today, according to many experts, almost every man diagnosed with prostate cancer might not even have cancer, and, even if he does, it is very likely to be progress very slowly, if it progresses at all. Thus, it is almost never justified to impose aggressive treatment especially on a man older than 75 or a man that has significant co-morbidities.

But, a man that walks into a urologists office with almost any kind of prostate problem should be aware that he is a "sitting duck" for a diagnosis of prostate cancer and subsequent treatment. This is especially true if he is the kind of guy that believes that "the only good cancer is the one that is cut out." Men and their partners that accept the immediate treatment mindset are almost invariably candidates for a radical prostatectomy.

Almost every doctor promotes treatments that he/she is most familiar with. The common high use of the radical prostatectomy reflects not that it is a better or best treatment, but that most practitioners that recommend it are also surgeons. Thus they are more familiar and comfortable with recommending surgery.

The bottom line is that – all treatments for prostate cancer have a similar profile of side effects. And, all induce a major deterioration in sexual satisfaction and ability. Some treatments, like a radical prostatectomy have side effects that are almost immediate, while others, like radiation, produce side effects weeks, months or even years later. But, I repeat this – all treatments for prostate cancer have life- altering side effects, regardless of what the medical provider says.

The Radical Prostatectomy

As mentioned above, the radical prostatectomy is the most common medical treatment for most men that receive a prostate cancer diagnosis. However, it is not the only treatment. Some men fall prone to the belief that other procedures may have less or more tolerable side effects. While it is true that the side effects vary for various treatments, it needs to be said loudly;

> **"All treatments for prostate cancer have serious side effects."**

While the radical prostatectomy is the most common treatment, it is a major surgery with a recovery time of about 4-6 weeks. It also carries general surgical risks of infection or complications. The major downside is that the surgery causes immediate erectile dysfunction and incontinence, both of which may be permanent.

Radiation and other prostate cancer treatments have similar side effects but they may be immediate or long-range. In any event, if a man, after extensive study and research, decides he needs treatment, he would be wise to seek out a professional that is not married to a specific procedure, but one the oversees the entire situation and evaluates it to the good of the patient, rather than to the good of his practice.

This is a strong statement and frequently a tough choice. Almost every urologist is trained as a surgeon and most recommend surgery to totally remove the prostate as the preferred treatment. Any man diagnosed with prostate cancer and facing a recommendation of a prostatectomy would be wise to check out the many articles from reputable sources and educate himself on the need for the procedure as well as seek a second opinion from an unconnected qualified authority.

Total surgical removal of the prostate gland, known as a radical prostatectomy is the most common choice for treating prostate cancer after diagnosis. With this procedure, the entire prostate gland plus some of the tissue and structures around it, including the seminal vesicles are removed.

The consequences of a radical prostatectomy are profound. Many of them relate to urinary and sexual function. However, one of the main considerations should be that recent research suggests that, for the majority of the cases, aggressive treatment may not really be needed.

A radical prostatectomy is a procedure touted by conventional medicine for curing prostate cancer. It has been performed for many years and is regarded as "gold standard" of prostate cancer treatment, although there are few studies that compare its efficacy to other techniques. It is a major pelvic surgery.

The prostate is located deep with the pelvis and there are many critical structures in close proximity to it. The surgery itself is technically formidable. Nearby structures include the urinary bladder and rectum. Damage to these structures during surgery can cause permanent disability. Nerve damage or trauma during surgery can lead to issues with ejaculation as well as erectile dysfunction and/or urinary as well as fecal incontinence.

Surgical damage to blood circulation can cause lasting disabilities. In the recent past, several surgeons have promoted nerve-sparing and bloodless techniques in an attempt to eliminate of minimize side effects. Other surgical risks are much the same as any other pelvic surgery and include, excessive bleeding at the surgical site, infection, and damage to ancillary organs.

Until recently, these side effects have not been relatively well-classified. Most side effects are those reported by urologists performing the surgery. This reporting, has been, in past years, rather poorly detailed and skimpy. Surgeons are not always particularly anxious to publicize the shortcomings of a procedure to which they have attached the "gold standard" label.

The most reported side effects are; erectile dysfunction and urinary incontinence. Unfortunately, even though reports have been filed, the bias of the doctors filing them is questionable. For example, a report detailing one of the major side effects, the problem of postoperative erectile dysfunction, ranges between 14 and 90 percent. This is a ludicrously wide range.

Based on my many years of practice, the published side effect statistics are a very optimistic estimate, likely provided by urologists that either do not want to admit their procedure causes such harm, or are in denial about the side effects and results.

In my practice, I have seen many men that were told by their urologist that they needed immediate treatment for their *prostate cancer.* Surgery was the usual option. Many of these guys opted not to have surgery. Some went for other treatments, like radiation, and others decided to find a practitioner that was amicable to watchful waiting. Most chose surgery. Those that decided on waiting, either went into a watchful waiting program under the auspices of their doctor or simply by themselves.

Often those choosing surgery are treating psychological fears more then cancer. Many doctors have a "doom and gloom" perspective when talking to their patients. If the patient is scared enough, he will likely do whatever the doctor recommends without much thought or questioning. Keeping the patient and his partner in the dark goes with the territory – especially regarding treatment side effects.

One of my clients related this story to me:

> "I was waiting in the hospital bed, prior to my surgery scheduled for the following morning. My doctor, a urologist, came in to check on me. I was very concerned about the possibility of erectile dysfunction, had spoken to my doctor about it several times, and had yet to receive a complete answer. I posed my question again, and his response was 'Well, we can visualize the erectile nerves very well.' I didn't press him further, but I should have. I had the surgery. The last time I had a natural erection was the day before that surgery five years ago."

This man had become my client after his radical prostatectomy. The surgery had left him totally and completely impotent. His sex drive and libido was intact. But, he was surprised that he could become extremely aroused sexually, and his arousal had absolutely no effect on his penis. He had come to me in the hope that I had some magical herbal remedies that would restore his sex life to what it was before the surgery.

At his request, we tried a few different herbals, but I told him at the outset, that I had little hope for success. As an interesting note, he was still consulting with the same urologist that performed his prostate sugery, only now, this same doctor was pushing him to have surgery again, this time for him to implant a penile prosthesis so he could get an artificial erection.

For these of you that are unfamiliar with a penile prosthesis, it is a device that is surgically implanted in the penis. It consists of two inflatable chambers that are inserted into the penis to replace the corpus cavernosum, the inflatable chambers of an intact penis that fill with blood to crease an erection. In my opinion, this is a last resort used only when nothing else can bring acceptable results. It has one serious drawback, – there is no way it can be undone if you are unhappy with it.

Making a long story short, I finally convinced him to change doctors. His new doctor, at my request had written him a prescription for synthetic prostaglandin called MisoProstol. A very low dose of this drug, introduced directly via his urethra, along with an over-the-counter vacuum erection device restored his ability to have an almost normal erection along with reestablishing a satisfying sexual relationship with his wife.

Albeit, he will never have a natural erection again due to the surgery, but what he has now is pretty close to natural, and has made both him and his wife quite happy. More detailed information about this technique is available in my book, "Solutions for Erectile Dysfunction." For a link to buy this book, visit my Facebook/James Occhiogrosso page.

I have found it extremely rare for a man that has had a radical prostatectomy to be satisfied with his postoperative erectile function, even after a period of years after the surgery. Similarly, urinary incontinence is a major issue. Most men experience a period of urinary incontinence after the surgery and some never regain complete continence.

Side effects of Other Prostate Treatments

All prostate cancer treatments have serious, life-altering side effects. Many men believe they can avoid such side effects by choosing a different treatment procedure. **They can not!** While the side effects of some procedures are immediate, others have side effects that creep-up tenuously over time.

For example: A radical prostatectomy removes the prostate as well as the seminal vesicles which provide the bulk of the ejaculate volume during an orgasm. Thus, a specific side effect of a radical prostatectomy is a dry orgasm.

Additionally, anorgasmia (inability to have an orgasm) is a frequent side effect of both radiation therapy as well as radical prostatectomy. Both treatments also have a high percentage of erectile dysfunction. In a Dec 2019 study, a lack of ejaculation was reported in up to 89% of patients that were treated with external beam radiation therapy. [10]

When I mention erectile dysfunction as a side effect of treatment, most men worry about it, but few really understand it. Almost every man suffers a bout of erectile dysfunction somewhere in his life. For most it is a temporary setback. However, there is a huge difference between an occasional bout of erectile dysfunction and the side effect of complete dysfunction due to treatment damage to the erectile nerves.

As a client who had total erectile dysfunction from radical prostatectomy related to me, – "I feel like I am no longer a man. Mentally, I get sexually aroused, but physically nothing happens. It is like my penis is totally dead."

Erectile dysfunction, lack of a satisfactory orgasm and incontinence seem to be the most concerning treatment side effects in the huge cohort of men that have been treated for prostate cancer.

However, they are not the only side effects reported. All treatments for prostate cancer can potentially include:

- Frequent, difficult or painful urination.
- Blood in the urine.
- Urinary leakage.
- Abdominal cramping.
- Diarrhea.
- Painful bowel movements.
- Rectal bleeding and/or stool leakage.
- Fatigue
- Sexual dysfunction
- Secondary cancers (radiation)
- Incontinence during sexual activity
- Nocturnal incontinence
- Painful or sensation-less orgasm
- Dry orgasm
- Anorgasmia
- Penile shrinkage (radical prostatectomy) – Removal of the prostate initiates a phase of penile shrinkage that varies between 2 to 3 cm

(approximately 1-2 inches). For men with large organs, this may have little effect, but a man that starts out on the small side, might be very dismayed about it.

Most doctors use PDE5 inhibitors (Viagra, Cialis, Levitra) to try to help rehabilitate patients with post surgery ED. However, success is not guaranteed. If the surgery has caused trauma or damage to the erectile nerves, it is unlikely that any of the PDE5 inhibitors will have a significant effect.

A 2011 study of 63 men that had undergone a radical prostatectomy found that about 75 percent of them sought treatment for erectile dysfunction. Additionally, more than 50 percent of the men reported having lower libido (sexual desire), and roughly an additional 40 percent were unable to have an orgasm or rate their orgasm as not satisfying [11]

The mental health effects of these symptoms were worse among highly sexually motivated participants. In fact, 52 percent reported that this had affected their self-esteem, and 36 percent reported having performance anxiety.

Additionally, there are few women that can tolerate urine leakage during sexual activity, as well as few men that can tolerate pain during intercourse. Many men have unrealistic expectations for sexual recovery after surgery. In my opinion, these unrealistic expectations are not countered by their doctors. All treatments for prostate cancer have permanent side effects.

Long-term permanent erectile dysfunction is a common consequence of a radical prostatectomy. This can be a huge issue for both a man and his partner. Many doctors are simply too busy or disinterested to spend much time explaining this common consequence of surgery.

Even when a man's doctor is quite candid with regard to reduced or non-existent sexual function, many men still expect improvements in sexual functioning, sometimes for years after surgery. Some men may recover usable erections after surgery. However, it is inevitable that sexual sensations after a prostate cancer treatment will never be the same as they were before. In most cases, sensation is greatly altered from what it was before. Therefore, if a patient's expectation for success means a recovery to the physical action and sensations prior to surgery, he is destined to be disappointed.

Loss of erectile function often causes a devastating blow to a man used to having sexual performance on demand for his entire life. Due to a lack of communication with his doctor, he may also be rather surprised about how total the loss is. This loss may also be perceived quite strongly by his partner.

Quite often, a man's partner can foster psychological feelings of rejection due to misunderstanding of the nature of erectile dysfunction due to surgery. Thus, it is important to bring explain the side effects of the surgery to the partner as well as the patient.

Since complete erectile dysfunction is a very real possibility after surgery, any man considering prostate treatment, surgery or otherwise should consider all other options very seriously, especially if he has a low grade Gleason 6 diagnosis. Surgery should be the last choice, not the first.

Watchful Waiting / Active Surveillance

A guy diagnosed with prostate cancer today has a multitude of choices. Unfortunately, considering the dynamic automobile analogy I discussed a few chapters before, getting a second opinion is not always a viable choice unless you know a urologist that is not hung up on doing surgery.

Active surveillance and watchful waiting are analogous terms referring to the process of holding back extensive treatment of a man diagnosed with prostate cancer, until such time as it appears the disease is appearing to progress to a more serious stage. I consider the terms interchangeable.

As of 2019, there were a little more than 13,000 practicing urologists in the US. About 90 percent of them are male. More than half are over the age of 55, while nearly 30 percent are aged 65 years or older. Thus, the vast majority of practicing urologists are older males.

Many of them are set in their ways and not terribly willing to change their practices drastically. The latest research on prostate cancer unanimously agrees that is over diagnosed and over treated, but not all urologists are willing to accept this fact.

I would venture an opinion that very few urologists dealing with prostate cancer today, have seriously looked at changing how they have treated their prostate cancers patients for years. For a urologist to accept foregoing the usual treatment in favor of active surveillance takes an open mind and many practicing older male urologists will not consider it.

Couple this with the fact that the vast majority of them are over 60, my opinion is that very few of them have taken the time to fully analyze and incorporate using active surveillance in their practice.

As a natural health practitioner, and herbologist, I have interfaced with many urologists over the years. I have met very few willing to accept that some herbal extracts can be very useful for their prostate patients. This apprehension of "anything natural" seems to be shared mostly by older practitioners. If they are willing to consider active surveillance at all, their definition is a PSA test and a prostate biopsy every few of months. In my opinion, if a man truly has a cancerous lesion in his prostate, this is just a way to wait for it to spread.

To me, active surveillance or watchful waiting is the time when dietary and lifestyle changes can make a huge difference. Even if the man does not truly have cancer, such changes can improve his health tremendously. Active surveillance can be viewed as a gift of time to rectify a bad situation in the body and improve ones overall health.

Many of the urologists I met were either unfamiliar with, or outright dismissed, herbal supplements used elsewhere in the world to effectively treat prostate conditions. Again, in my opinion, this *closed mind* attitude is detrimental to their patients.

A 2009 Cochrane database review concluded that "The evidence suggests that Saw Palmetto (Seronoa repens provides mild to moderate improvement in urinary symptoms and flow. It also produced similar improvement in urinary symptoms and flow when compared with the prescription drug, finasteride. and is associated with fewer adverse treatment events."

Active surveillance is the process of monitoring a patient with a diagnosis of gland-confined low-risk prostate cancer over time to try and improve the cancer situation without having any progression.

Some medical practitioners view active surveillance as the process of waiting for the cancer to indicate it is spreading. They are anticipating progression so additional aggressive treatment can be initiated. Thus, the gift of time given to them by nature is simply a way to placate patients. The patient is steeped in the belief that his disease is being carefully watched, but it is a false belief. Most cancers are the result of a failed immune process. And, if the elements that caused the cancer to originally appear are not changed, the cancer is likely to grow or spread.

A far better approach is to use well researched natural techniques to limit the potential spread of the disease by improving the overall health of the body and its immune system. This is where active surveillance becomes truly active. Instead of simply remeasuring the PSA every six (or so) months and following the usual PSA guidelines for a biopsy, truly active surveillance consists of using herbal extracts, changes in dietary habits, lifestyle changes, as well as various vitamins and other nutrients.

Prostate specific herbal supplements have been used successfully worldwide for hundreds of years. The goal of active surveillance is to alter the conditions that caused the cancer. By altering conditions towards a more healthy environment, the body has the opportunity to activate its immune power to destroy or shrink the cancer.

Studies show that many men opting for a truly active surveillance, go for many years will little progression of their cancer and no aggressive medical attention needed. Since this condition develops mostly among older men, it tends to allow the man to die from other causes. Thus, a man, diagnosed with prostate cancer, may live out his life *with* prostate cancer rather than die from it.

More holistic medical practitioners as well as naturopaths view this time period as a gift to allow time for natural processes to work. Cancer occurs because of the inability of the body's immune system to destroy wayward cells like it should. A holistic approach to active surveillance means that the waiting period between active testing is a period whereby one has an opportunity to slow down or beat the disease.

> Also, a man with diagnosed low-risk prostate cancer can use active surveillance for many years. It generally means a few, potentially welcome changes must be made in his life. And, it is an approach that does not destroy his sexual ability or otherwise complicate his life. [12]

Non-Cancerous Problems

As a man ages, prostate problems become more frequent and often, more troublesome. Medically, many of these issues are referred to urologists for treatment. Some are more serious than others. However, of the problems listed below, none are expected to lead to cancer, the most serious prostate problem.

For many men, this is their biggest fear and an unscrupulous practitioner can pick up on it. For the record, if you get nothing else out of this book, know that **none** of the problems listed in this section lead to prostate cancer, regardless of what your doctor says.

During many years of practice, I was stunned several times by a client mentioning to me that his/her doctor said that treatment was necessary before the condition turned into cancer. I use both genders here, because I heard this issue from both male and female clients. Men with either prostatitis or BPH were told they needed immediate treatment, as well as were perimenopausal women with painful uterine fibroids.

In both cases, they were told that their condition would turn into cancer if they did not deal with it immediately. This is a blatant scare tactic, since there is no evidence whatsoever that either condition leads to cancer

While this book is primarily directed towards men, I was privileged to help many woman as well. The typical scenario for a woman was that she was menopausal or entering menopause, and was having pain that often mimicked the cramps and pain she used to have when her menses was active. This is quite common for late forties women, and is often an indicator of uterine or ovarian fibroid tumors. It is not an indication of cancer.

The tumors tend to grow during or after menopause, in a manner similar to the prostate growth a man experiences with aging. At certain times of the month, the fibroids can be painful and some women consult with a urologist to resolve them. The visit typically results in various scans before the diagnosis of fibroid tumors is made.

In many cases, the words tumor is critical in the woman's mind. Like a man, she is fearful and wary of cancer. Statistics for uterine and ovarian cancer have been drummed into her mind for years and she likely has had a relative or friend that succumbed to the disease over the years. Again, this is a condition that is ripe for an unscrupulous practitioner to take advantage of.

During my practice, I consulted with several woman that were told they needed a hysterectomy, a procedure that surgically removes the woman's uterus, and often her ovaries. In many cases, the woman was told she needed to have the surgery as soon as possible, before it turned into cancer.

Like men, women also fear the dreaded cancer diagnosis. Like men, they are also bombarded by media about early treatment preventing a disaster. Like men, they are vulnerable to the suggestion that their treatment needs to include surgery to prevent the cancer from going further and destroying their lives. Like men, many of them succumb to the practitioner's advice and agree to surgery. And, like men, they suffer the side effects of the surgery for the rest of their lives. klotsz

Other Non-Cancerous Prostate and Urinary Issues

I have devoted this book to helping guys avoid the disaster of a prostate cancer diagnosis and subsequent aggressive treatment. However, there are many other problems that befall the aging man and his reproductive parts. These are listed below. Note that none of the leads to, or is indicative of, prostate cancer.

• **Prostate Enlargement** – As I mentioned in the beginning, the male prostate is the only organ in the body that tends to enlarge with aging. This enlargement is called Benign Prostate Hyperplasia (or Hypertrophy or more commonly, BPH). It is a non-cancerous growth of tissue in the prostate.

> BPH can cause a host of problems for a man, mostly in the area of urination issues. While it does contribute to problems like erectile dysfunction and disruption of urination, there is no evidence it leads to prostate cancer. However, it is quite possible the two conditions can coexist in the same man.

• **Prostatitis** – This is a condition where the prostate is irritated or inflamed. Its cause can be either a bacterial infection, general inflammation or unknown. It can cause pain and swelling around the pelvic area and is often treated with antibiotics like Cipro.

> With regard to Cipro – this is a rather strong antibiotic with a host of side effects. I have seen several clients that were put on Cipro for prostatitis without first determining that their condition was bacterial. In my opinion, this is simply bad medical practice.

Many men (and a few women) have developed serious tendon tears when Cipro or a similar antibiotic was prescribed. This is a documented, and well-known side effect of this class of antibiotics. If a drug like Cipro is used, it should only be used for a confirmed active bacterial infection. It should not be used as a general cookie-cutter treatment for any man that is complaining of pelvic pain.

Prostatitis can be initiated by stress or several kinds of activity. Motorcycle, bike and horseback riding, as well as rough sex tend to put physical stress on the pelvic area and can initiate prostatitis. The condition often self-resolves after a period of rest.

I have consulted with several male clients that had a sudden large jump in their PSA results. In many cases, their PSA returned to a normal or near normal value as soon as the stress element was eliminated. Males that have sex with other males (especially on the receiving end) often have a rise in PSA for a few days after the encounter. This should trigger a few days of rest, but if the examiner is a urologist, it often triggers an order for a prostate biopsy.

• **Urinary Tract Infections (UTI's)** – Common with both men and women, a UTI can result in a high degree of pain, inability to urinate normally, serious discomfort, and, in a man, an elevated PSA. A UTI is almost always initiated by a bacterial infection and is generally treated with some kind of antibiotic.

Some people are prone to getting them. When this is the case, it is prudent for the patient to see a nutritionist or a naturopath to determine why a UTI was produced. Successive courses of antibiotics usually cause more problems then they solve. For someone prone to these issues a long-term course of a natural antibiotic such as; Colloidal Silver or Oregano Oil combined with a few dietary changes may help.

There are many other problems that can result from unhealthy dietary and lifestyle habits. Many of them effect the reproduction system. One of the reasons for this is that the reproduction system, especially in the area of erectile dysfunction is highly dependent on good blood circulation.

Many men have used PDE-3 drugs similar to Viagra to help with the inability to generate or sustain an erection. A satisfactory sexual erection is a combination of many factors in the hormonal system and is strongly dependent upon good blood circulation. Arteries in the penile area are not unique. If they are blocked enough to prevent a normal erection, you can be sure that there are blockages in other arteries as well.

Please note that the above is, by no means, a complete listing of all of the problems that can befall the male prostate, urinary and sexual system. The three issues above are simply the most common aging-type issues men face that result in them seeing a medical professional. There is a wealth of information available on the Internet about each of these conditions.

Resolving the Urinary issues of BPH with a TURP

For some men, long term BPH is often relieved with a procedure called a Trans-Urethral Prostatectomy or a TURP. This procedure removes prostate tissue by passing a cutting instrument through the penis to the prostate. It is usually done to relieve blockage from the excess prostate tissue and allow better urination.

While it is still a surgical procedure, subject to the usual risks of surgery, it is a lessor procedure than a prostatectomy, and, for younger men, can often solve urinary problems. However, I have had several clients, mostly in the mid to late 80′s that have done poorly with this procedure due to their age and co-morbidities. (See section on self-catheterization below)

A TURP is a procedure used to enhance the flow of urine for men that have BPH slowing their urine stream significantly. For younger men, It is an effective treatment for urinary symptoms, especially urinary retention due to BPH, but it is still surgery with all the attendant surgical risks and potential complications

The TURP is most useful for younger men. It allows the majority of patients to void acceptably afterwards without severe consequences. However, in the older male, (over 80) it is associated with significant morbidity.

Urologists often recommend a TURP for almost every man that presents with urinary difficulties and enlarged prostate due to BPH.

Aside from the usual surgical complications, a TURP may have long term effects that are permanent. The common ones are:

- Permanent injury to the bladder or the bladder sphincter muscle resulting in incontinence.

- Excessive post-operative bleeding or blood in the urine.

- Electrolyte imbalance lasting beyond the procedure.

- Infection.

- Loss of erections.

- Painful or difficult urination.

Retrograde ejaculation is almost always a side effect of a TURP. This occurs because most of the ejaculate goes backwards into the bladder rather then out of the penis. Aside from its emotional impact retrograde ejaculation is not harmful (unless you are planning to make babies). It has little effect on orgasm.

> Postoperative bleeding may last for 3 to 4 weeks after the procedure. It is usually directly related to the size of the BPH-swollen-gland and duration of the procedure. A urinary catheter is usually placed in the bladder for a short period after surgery. The surgery typically lasts about 90 minutes and the catheter is usually removed within 1-2 days. [13]

Urinary Self-Catheterization

Men over 80 years old may have a hard time recovering from a TURP, especially if they are relatively weak or have co-morbidities. Although few urologists push self-catheterization, in my opinion, it is better to have these men learn to use this approach rather than subject them to the strain of TURP surgery.

A men that is familiar with a catheter probably gained his familiarity in a hospital emergency room at 3 am. Older men with BPH tend to experience urinary blockage in the early morning hours. The hospital experience is often their first introduction to a catheter and a collection bag. It is also fair to say they were somewhat traumatized by the situation.

Acute urinary retention typically occurs to a man during the night-time hours, and he usually winds up in the emergency room (ER), painfully waiting for someone to catheterize him to alleviate the over-pressure situation in his bladder. A catheter, (called a Foley catheter, after its inventor) is typically inserted in the ER by a nurse, immediately relieving the acute stress on the kidneys and the bladder. When the man is released from the ER, (with the catheter and a collection bag in place), he is told to make a follow-up appointment with a urologist.

A Foley catheter is a cumbersome device consisting of tubes for collecting the urine and an inflatable balloon for retaining itself in the bladder. The practitioner must pass the mechanism through the man's penis and prostate and into the bladder. When the end is passed into the bladder, and urine is flowing, the small balloon is inflated with saline solution to anchor the catheter in place. The tubes passed through the penis are relatively thick and undoubtedly cause pain and discomfort as they are passed in.

For many men, this is where a downward roller coaster slide begins. The lucky guy keeps the catheter in for a few days to a week or so, then goes to the urologist, gets it removed and is able to urinate normally again. The unlucky guy gets the catheter removed, still can't urinate, and shortly afterward gets it put back in, often the same day at the same visit. This is typically when he is advised that a biopsy is needed!

The bottom line is that there are many ways to alleviate the urinary retention issues associated with BPH. Any man that has such issues would be wise to see a natural health professional while these issues are just mildly annoying before he finds himself in a medical emergency situation, rushing to the ER at 3 am with a painfully full urinary bladder, or undergoing a surgical procedure.

Self catheterization is considerably simpler and painless. Since it is used only for the time it takes to void and then removed, it does not need the bulky mechanism of the retention balloon or the collection bag that is inherently part of a Foley catheter. Thus, a self-catheter can be considerably thinner. It is simply a piece of plastic tubing, long enough to pass through the penis and to the bladder and thin enough to be painlessly fed through the urethra and the penis. Self-catheters can be obtained in single-use form or reusable as well as many thicknesses. The reusable form should be cleaned thoroughly with soap and water after each use.

> Older men usually find the self-catheterization to be very simple and easy to implement. Most quickly become comfortable doing it and a catheter can simply be coiled up and slipped into a pants pocket for away from home activities. The urine output is directed into the toilet as if it were the man's normal urine stream. [14]

For older men or men with co-morbidities that prohibit a TURP with all its attendant side effects, self-catheterization is a viable and safe alternative. For more information see the reference below. [15]

Personal Action Items

With the exception of a brief mention of the herb Saw Palmetto ((Seronoa repens) in a chapter above, I have deliberately avoided making nutritional or herbal supplement recommendations in this book. There is a wealth of information about various supplements and nutritional items that can help a man dealing with low-risk prostate cancer. Unfortunately, in today's electronic age, anyone can say almost anything they like about a product, and, as long as they do not violate any of the FDA's general rules, promote almost any product they like.

In this book, I have devoted my effort mainly to the guy that unconsciously views his doctor as the bearer of the last word on everything related to his prostate issue. In a chapter above, I related the story of one of my clients that had had multiple prostate biopsies due to a lump on his prostate that was likely congenital. It highlights the case of a doctor that just does not care much about patient suffering and a patient that accepts anything the doc says without enganging his mind.

Another case is the one where the doctor does not actually know about other possible treatments for his patient. This is illustrated by a situation I found myself in several years ago. A urologist at a meeting I was attending knew I was an herbalist and asked if I knew anything about Saw Palmetto. At first, I though he was fooling around, but as we talked further, I realized he knew nothing about the herb. I gave him a brief dissertation about it, but after the initial sentence or two, I think he lost interest. What amazed me about this sad encounter was that this guy was a practicing urologist, and, he knew nothing about an herb that is a mainstay of prostate treatment worldwide.

Any guy that wants some specific recommendations might be well served to get a copy of my book, *"Your Prostate, Your Libido, Your Life"* where I review almost 500 clinical studies of various herbal and nutritional items that are known to be useful for male prostate health. It is available through a link to the GoodReads site from my facebook page, "Facebook/James Occhiogrosso."

This brings me to my list of items that any man dealing with prostate issues should be aware of before he submits to any kind of treatment:

• Know your doctor and his mindset. If your doctor is the kind of person that cannot ever be wrong, perhaps someone that is more vulnerable – and – open to new ideas would be a better choice..

• Read your doctors published material. If material published for a procedure he promotes highlights only the benefits and is silent about any side effects, beware.

• Ask questions you already know the answers for. If you have BPH and you ask your doctor to expand on that, and he gives you a dissertation about how it leads to prostate cancer, find another doctor.

• Read, learn and question. – Most doctors say they welcome questions from patients, but, do they really? Many only welcome questions that fit in with their treatment paradigm. Ask questions about well-known supplements. If your doctor is unaware of them, or immediately disparages all supplements, ask why. If you don't get a solid answer back, it is time to find another doctor.

• Do not be fooled by the slick advertisements for supplements on TV, especially those on late night TV. As I said above, anyone can say almost anything, and most of these late night ads usually do. While there are many valuable supplements that can be used, few that are well-researched and effective will be found on late-night TV.

- If you are planning a watchful waiting approach, find a holistic practitioner to guide you in choosing your nutritional or herbal supplements.

Most of all, unless you have implicit trust in your medical practitioner, do not agree to any aggressive treatment without fully researching it. And, this means more than just asking some friends on the golf course or at the gym. Research takes time.

Conclusions and Discussion

The main question I pose in this book is about the current medical diagnosis and treatment of prostate cancer. Is such a diagnosis and its associated treatment actually helping men live a longer and better life, or is it creating a disaster where none existed before. Are we fixing a problem or creating one?

Trying to answer this question with research on the Internet indicates there is a paucity of studies that examine what happens when men diagnosed with prostate cancer avoid or refuse treatment. In addition, many of the studies actually published were written by urologists that treat prostate cancer and are often biased towards the treatments they provide.

The cookie-cutter approach used by many urologists today is seriously not working. It seems to be the result of an overwhelmed cadre of physicians that simply accept the status-quo. I hope this book can shed some light on it for the average older man.

According to the medical community, it would be unethical to promote a study where conventional treatment would be withheld for some patients. However, such a study was performed in 2008 comparing arthroscopic knee surgery (the conventional treatment) with a placebo.

Critics from the medical profession (generally orthopedic surgeons) screamed and hollered that this was an unethical study because it denied the usual conventional (proven, gold standard, etc.) treatment to patients. The conclusion of this study is below:

"Arthroscopic surgery for osteoarthritis of the knee provides no additional benefit to optimized physical and medical therapy."[16] *Link # 16*

Traditionally, surgery is often based on guidelines, protocols and educated guessing rather than solid scientific data. When a questionable surgery is properly compared to a placebo (a sham surgery), the results are often surprising and generate much controversy – especially among practitioners whose livelihood is significantly dependent on such surgery.

To the best of my knowledge, there has been no rigorous studies that compare patients diagnosed with Gleason 6 prostate cancer with other forms of prostate cancer or diagnosed but not medically treated.

According to some experts, what is currently defined as Gleason 6 prostate cancer may not even be prostate cancer. It is often an indolent process and does not usually spread. However, patients diagnosed with Gleason 6 prostate cancer are routinely subjected to surgical treatment with a radical prostatectomy. Any proposed study that would clarify this will inevitably be subject to loud voices that it is unethical.

But then, my question is: – is it ethical to treat men for a disease they do not really have, especially considering that the treatment will likely permanently reduce their quality of life and destroy their sexual life?

Institutional corruption and individual greed have, for the past 2 to 3 decades hampered progress in prostate cancer diagnosis and management. Unfortunately, until the public becomes aware of this, any man facing a prostate cancer diagnosis, especially a Gleason 6 diagnosis, is in dangr of having his sexuality terminated. This is, of course, unless he chooses a practitioner that is not dedicated to dubious practices designed to enrich the connected few with little regard to the damage left behind.

I am not an advocate of bashing the medical profession, but I do recognize that for nearly three decades after the approval of the PSA as a test for prostate cancer by the FDA, several thousand men have had their prostates removed unnecessarily. Many of these men lost their sexuality even though they were in a very low-risk category and might have lived with the condition for many years.

The PSA test was invented by Dr. Richard Ablin, who says it never should have been put into use as a diagnostic test for prostate cancer. In a 2014 interview Dr. Ablin was quoted as saying many men will develop prostate cancer by age 70. If an older man has a PSA level that prompts a biopsy, it is likely you will find cancer. In the 2008 autopsy study quoted above, Dr. Haas found that the incidence of indolent prostate cancer to be about equivalent, percentage wise, to the man's age. To put this another perhaps clearer, way,

If you are 70 years old, you likely have a 70 percent chance of having prostate cancer.

So, is this cancer that is offering you no symptoms, the one you want to give up the rest of your sexual life for?

I have come to the conclusion in the recent past, that, in many cases, doctors are in denial about the pain and suffering caused by unneeded medical tests and procedures. There needs to be a hard look at how prostate cancer is diagnosed and treated. And, this look should involve unbiased medical researchers without embedded financial connections.

This is not to minimize the effects of aggressive prostate cancer. It can spread to the lymph nodes[1] of the pelvis or throughout the body. Advanced prostate cancer often tends to spread to the bones in the pelvis causing severe pain and often resulting in death. However, the bulk of prostate treatment usually involves men that have not been seriously evaluated for low-risk, indolent prostate cancer. They are often subjected to surgery, radiation or other treatments that leave them feeling like they are part of "the walking dead" rather than cancer survivors!

---

1. https://www.cancer.gov/Common/PopUps/popDefinition.aspx?id=CDR0000045762&version=Patient&language=English

REFERENCES

[1]Bloodletting—https://en.wikipedia.org/wiki/Bloodletting

[2]Key Statistics for Prostate Cancer, American Cancer Society, 2021

[3]Gabriel P Haas, Et al, The worldwide epidemiology of prostate cancer: perspectives from autopsy studies,

Can J Urol, 2008 Feb;15(1):3866-71.

[4]Dr. Bert Vorstman, The Robotic Prostate Cancer Surgery Nightmare, Urology Web blog, Florida Urological Associates

[5]Oregon Health & Science University. "Presence Of High-risk Prostate Cancer Can Be Predicted Without A Biopsy, New Study Says." ScienceDaily. ScienceDaily, 22 May 2005.

[6]Howard Wolinsky, Is This Really Cancer? Movement builds to classify Gleason 6 prostate lesions as nonmalignant, MedPage Today, January 9, 2021

[7]Mark Stolz, MD, et al, What Is Gleason 6 Prostate Cancer?, Very Wellhealth Blog, August 02, 2021

[8]Samantha Bonar, Emotional Impact of Prostate Cancer, City of Hope blog, March 9, 2017

[9]Richard M. Hoffman, et al, Treatment Decision Regret Among Long-Term Survivors of Localized Prostate Cancer: Results From the Prostate Cancer Outcomes Study, Journal of Clinical Oncology, Vol. 35, No. 20, July 10, 2017

[10]Travis P. Green, et al, Ejaculatory and Orgasmic Dysfunction Following Prostate Cancer Therapy: Clinical Management, Journal List, Med Sci (Basel), v.7(12); 2019 Dec

[11]O.Bratu, et al, Erectile dysfunction post-radical prostatectomy – a challenge for both patient and physician, J Med Life., 2017 Jan-Mar; 10(1): 13–18.

[12]Laurence Klotz,MD, et al, Long-Term Follow-Up of a Large Active Surveillance Cohort of Patients With Prostate Cancer, American Society of Clinical Oncology,J Clin Oncol 33:272-277. 2014

[13]Olapade-Olaopa, MD, et al, Haematuria and clot retention after transurethral resection of the prostate: a pilot study, Department of Urology, Leicester General Hospital, Gwendolen Road, Leicester LE5 4PW, UK. 07 July 2008

[14]R.D. Brierly, et al, Is transurethral resection of the prostate safe and effective in the over 80-year-old?, Ann R Coll Surg Engl, 2001 Jan;83(1):50-3.

[15]Sloan Kettering Institute, Self-Catheterization for Males, Patient & Caregiver Education, January 6, 2021

*[16]*Alexandra Kirkley, M.D., et al, A Randomized Trial of Arthroscopic Surgery for Osteoarthritis of the Knee, N Engl J Med 2008; 359:1097-1107, September 11, 2008.

Don't miss out!

Visit the website below and you can sign up to receive emails whenever James Occhiogrosso publishes a new book. There's no charge and no obligation.

https://books2read.com/r/B-A-AOZG-DFSPB

BOOKS 2 READ

Connecting independent readers to independent writers.

Also by James Occhiogrosso

Solutions for Erectile Dysfunction
Your Prostate, Your Libido, Your Life
Dr. Jim's Guide to the Aging Male Body
Dr. Jim's Guide to Avoiding a Prostate Nightmare

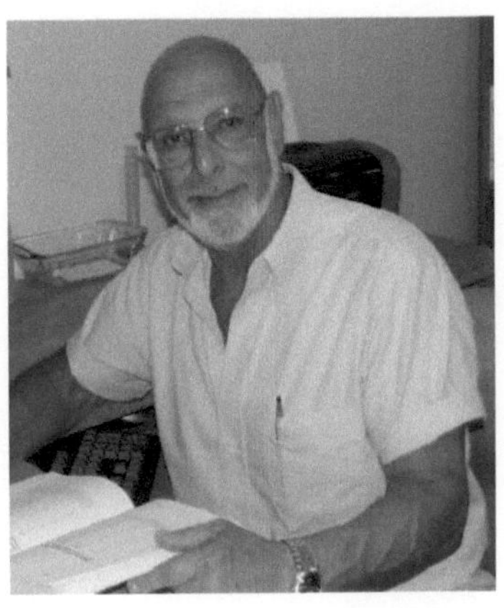

About the Author

James Occhiogrosso, N.D. is a Natural Health Practitioner specializing in male and female health issues and author of "Your Prostate, Your Libido, Your Life" and "Solutions for Erectile Dysfunction." He maintains an active practice helping both men and women overcome hormonal and sexual issues associated with aging, including loss of libido, erectile dysfunction and menopausal issues, and often acts as an advisor for men with prostate cancer whose doctors recommend a "watchful waiting" approach. Salivary home hormone test kits as well as bio-identical hormone creams are available at his website

He lives with his wife of nearly 40 years in Southwest Florida, USA

Connect with him at: DrJim@HealthNaturallyToday.com

OR

Facebook/James Occhiogrosso

www.ingramcontent.com/pod-product-compliance
Ingram Content Group UK Ltd.
Pitfield, Milton Keynes, MK11 3LW, UK
UKHW040030200726
13854UKWH00001B/455

9 798201 481117